Moxibustion for Fertility

Using Moxa Throughout Your Cycle to Improve Fertility, AHM,FSH, Ovarian Function and PCOS at Home

Dan Phillips PhD

~DEDICATION~

~LARRY~

For your unwavering support, encouragement, and friendship. Your presence in my life has been a constant source of inspiration. Thank you for your invaluable kindness and belief in my journey. This book is a token of appreciation for your enduring friendship and steadfast encouragement.

TABLE OF CONTENT

CHAPTER 1

Understanding Moxibustion for Fertility

A key element of traditional Chinese medicine (TCM), moxibustion is a healing method with a long history and a broad range of uses that has withstood the test of time. Its possible contribution to improving fertility has attracted more research and attention in recent years. This chapter provides a thorough overview of the age-old method of moxibustion and its applicability to enhancing fertility. Through an exploration of the historical background and basic concepts of moxibustion therapy, readers will get a more profound comprehension of its possible advantages for those aiming to enhance their reproductive process.

Moxibustion's Historical Origins and Development:

Moxibustion, also known as "jiu" in Chinese, has its roots in ancient China and dates back thousands of years. It was initially recorded in the founding text of Traditional Chinese Medicine (TCM), the "Huangdi Neijing" (Yellow Emperor's Inner Canon), an ancient medical literature. Moxibustion has been used historically to treat a variety of illnesses, such as pain management, immune system support, and reproductive health. Moxibustion's historical development demonstrates its versatility and effectiveness in a range of medical settings.

The Fundamental Ideas of Moxibustion:

The fundamental idea behind moxibustion's effectiveness is that it works by stimulating particular body locations to encourage the flow of blood and Qi, or life energy. The practice of carefully burning processed mugwort (Artemisia vulgaris), sometimes called as "moxa," produces this excitement. Moxa can be applied topically, such on the skin, directly (direct moxibustion) or indirectly (indirect moxibustion), by putting it on top of something like salt or ginger. Applying moxibustion produces heat, which is thought to support the body's innate healing processes.

In the context of reproduction, the basic ideas of moxibustion become even more important. Moxibustion employs specific acupuncture sites linked to hormone balance and reproductive organs to tackle underlying abnormalities that may impact fertility. This method is consistent with TCM's holistic approach to health, which holds that the body's interrelated systems have an impact on one another.

Fertility Enhancement and Moxibustion:

TCM's comprehension of the body's energy channels and their significance in reproductive health is the basis for the idea that moxibustion might improve fertility. Difficulties with conception may arise from disturbances in the circulation of Qi and blood, according to TCM philosophy. Moxibustion aims to produce the ideal conditions for conception and pregnancy by encouraging the efficient circulation of these essential chemicals.

The effects of moxibustion on fertility have been studied, and the findings are encouraging. According to studies, moxibustion may benefit ovarian function, uterine blood flow, and hormone balance, among other things. For example, moxibustion has been linked to increased blood flow to the ovaries and uterus, which may facilitate the formation and implantation of follicles.

Traversing the Contemporary Terrain:

The incorporation of moxibustion into methods for enhancing fertility is becoming more popular in the modern world. When people look into non-invasive and possibly beneficial methods to improve their reproductive health, moxibustion is one such choice. Furthermore, moxibustion techniques are a viable option for individuals who want more control over their reproductive journey because they are easily accessible for self-administration at home.

It's crucial to remember that, despite its potential, moxibustion is not a stand-alone treatment. Numerous factors affect fertility, such as nutrition, stress, lifestyle, and health issues. Moxibustion need to be seen as an adjunctive strategy that works in concert with other interventions to promote general well-being and reproductive objectives.

Conclusion

Upon exploring the nexus between conventional wisdom and contemporary science, the age-old modality of moxibustion presents itself as an intriguing means of boosting fertility. We set the stage for an in-depth examination of its applications in later chapters by comprehending its basic concepts and historical foundation. Further exploration of the field of moxibustion for fertility will reveal the precise means by which this traditional method can aid in the fulfillment of reproductive goals in the modern era.

CHAPTER 2

Moxibustion Techniques and Tools: Delve into the various techniques and tools used in moxibustion therapy for fertility. Discuss different types of moxa, such as direct and indirect, and how to select the appropriate method for different fertility-related conditions.

The ancient Chinese treatment known as moxibustion has become more well-known due to its claims to improve reproductive health and fertility. With this age-old method, heat is applied to particular acupuncture points on the body, mostly by burning a material called "moxa." We shall delve into the complex world of moxibustion methods and equipment utilized in reproductive therapies in this chapter. We'll explore the several kinds of moxa, like direct and indirect, and how they can be customized to treat specific issues linked to infertility.

Comprehension of Moxibustion:

Moxibustion has a 5,000-year history and is derived from the Chinese phrase "jiu," which means flaming plant. It is thought to encourage blood and Qi (vital energy) flow, fostering harmony and balance in the body. By treating underlying imbalances, enhancing blood flow to the reproductive organs, and fostering an environment that is favorable to conception, moxibustion is used to optimize reproductive function in the setting of fertility.

Moxibustion Types:

Moxibustion procedures can be broadly classified into two categories: direct and indirect.

1. Moxibustion Direct: A little moxa cone or cylinder is ignited and applied directly to the skin or an acupuncture point in direct moxibustion. Deeply penetrating the acupuncture point, the heat generated stimulates the flow of Qi and blood. There are two types of

direct moxibustion: scarring and non-scarring. By burning the moxa until it produces localized blistering and scarring, a technique known as "scarring moxibustion" frequently produces more potent medicinal effects. Removing the moxa before it burns the skin is necessary for non-scarring moxibustion.

2. Moxibustion Indirectly: In order to avoid direct heat contact, an intermediary such as ginger slices, salt, or aconite is placed between the skin and the moxa during indirect moxibustion. Light the moxa and hold it above the medium

to create a soft, non-burning heat that is sent to the acupuncture point. Since indirect moxibustion is said to be gentler than direct moxibustion, it is appropriate for people who have sensitive skin or who would rather take a more delicate approach.

Selecting the Correct Approach:

Choosing the right moxibustion technique for various fertility-related issues necessitates a thorough comprehension of the patient's constitution, diagnosis, and intended course of treatment.

While selecting between direct and indirect moxibustion, keep the following things in mind:

1. Sensitivity and Constitution: Direct moxibustion may be advantageous for people with thicker skin and strong constitutions. However, because indirect moxibustion lowers the possibility of skin irritation, people with thin or delicate skin may find it more appropriate.

2. Level of Severity: The higher stimulation of direct moxibustion may be chosen for extreme cases of

infertility. For ailments like hormonal imbalances or blocked fallopian tubes, it can have a stronger curative effect.

3. Static Situations: Long-term reproductive issues may benefit from indirect moxibustion, which gradually stimulates the body in a steady and mild manner. It is very helpful for treating underlying imbalances and controlling menstrual cycles.

4. Choosing an Acupuncture Point: The selection of moxibustion technique is also influenced by the

choice of acupuncture points. Because of their unique impacts on reproductive health, some points are better suited for direct moxibustion, while others might work better with indirect moxibustion.

Applications and Methods:

Practitioners use a variety of instruments and methods in addition to the type of moxibustion to improve the effectiveness of fertility-focused treatments:

1. Rolls of Moxa: Crushed moxa is used to make the cylindrical sticks known as moxa rolls. For indirect heating, they can be lit and held near the acupuncture sites. With their versatility, moxa rolls can be used for moxibustion in two ways: directly and indirectly.

2. Cones of Moxa: Moxa cones are tiny, cone-shaped moxa pieces that are applied topically to the skin for moxibustion. They work particularly well when precisely aiming at certain points.

3. Boxes Molxa: Moxa boxes are containers made to safely store burning moxa cones so that the smoke and heat may reach the acupuncture point. They offer a precise and concentrated application of heat.

4. Oxygen Sticks: Moxa sticks are used in indirect moxibustion; they have a cigar-like appearance. They have a soft, warming sensation when held over the skin or acupuncture points.

5. Heating lamps: Heat lamps are occasionally employed in

contemporary moxibustion procedures to deliver regulated and even heat to bigger regions, which helps to improve blood circulation.

Rendering:

The use of moxibustion instruments and procedures can improve fertility in a comprehensive way that is consistent with the principles of traditional Chinese medicine. The individual's condition, constitution, and treatment objectives should be taken into consideration while deciding between direct and indirect moxibustion and the right equipment. Consultation with a qualified and experienced practitioner is crucial, just as with any medical intervention. They can tailor moxibustion therapy to target certain fertility-related issues, ultimately enhancing reproductive health and general well-being.

CHAPTER 3

Optimizing Hormonal Balance with Moxibustion: Explore the relationship between moxibustion and hormonal balance. Examine how moxibustion can influence hormones like AHM (Anti-Mullerian Hormone) and FSH (Follicle-Stimulating Hormone) to improve fertility outcomes.

Hormonal homeostasis is a key component in the complex web of fertility, directing the reproductive processes in a nuanced dance. The importance of hormones like follicle-stimulating hormone (FSH) and anti-mullerian hormone (AMH) in relation to fertility has been clarified by recent developments in reproductive medicine. This chapter explores the intriguing relationship between hormonal balance and moxibustion therapy, revealing how moxibustion may improve fertility results by affecting these important hormones.

The Hormone Dance: Comprehending FSH and AMH:

A hormone called anti-Mullerian hormone (AMH) is a marker of ovarian reserve, or the amount of eggs left in a woman's ovaries. Essentially, it offers information about future reproductive potential. Conversely, the growth of follicles and ovulation depend heavily on the hormone called follicle-stimulating hormone (FSH).

Decreased ovarian function may be indicated by elevated FSH levels.

In the field of traditional Chinese medicine (TCM), hormonal equilibrium is said to be supported by the balance of Qi and blood. Reproductive health may be impacted by abnormalities in hormones that arise from disruptions in this equilibrium. As a method based on encouraging the movement of blood and Qi, moxibustion has the capacity to correct these imbalances.

Moxibustion and Hormone Harmonization:

Studies indicate that moxibustion could potentially regulate hormones such as FSH and AMH. In order to bring the endocrine system back into balance, moxibustion targets particular acupuncture sites linked to hormone regulation. Moxibustion is believed to produce localized heat that stimulates blood flow, which may have an impact on hormone secretion and production.

Research examining the effect of moxibustion on levels of AMH has produced some interesting findings. Preliminary results indicate that moxibustion may help maintain adequate levels of ovarian reserve, however more research is required. Likewise, studies examining the connection between moxibustion and FSH suggest that moxibustion may influence FSH levels, hence promoting the growth of healthy follicles.

Steering Through the Complexity: Tailored Methods:

Recognizing the complexity and individual heterogeneity of hormonal balance is crucial. There are many different causes of infertility, and no two people have the same hormonal composition. Within the comprehensive framework of Traditional Chinese Medicine, moxibustion acknowledges the individuality of every person's constitution and works to bring balance back on a case-by-case basis.

It is crucial to use moxibustion under the supervision of a licensed healthcare provider when thinking about using it to improve hormonal balance. An expert practitioner is able to determine any imbalances, evaluate each person's unique hormonal profile, and adjust moxibustion regimens accordingly. This customized method guarantees that moxibustion is used in a way that complements each person's particular requirements and reproductive objectives.

Beyond Hormones: A Comprehensive Approach:

Although hormonal balance is the main topic of this chapter, it is important to see moxibustion within a more comprehensive holistic framework. One aspect of moxibustion's complex impacts on the body is its capacity to affect hormones. Through the treatment of hormonal imbalances, moxibustion provides a holistic approach to improving fertility by increasing relaxation, lowering stress levels, and improving overall well-being.

In summary:

Hormones play a dual role in the complex process of fertility, acting as both messengers and architects in determining the trajectory of conception and pregnancy. With its origins in conventional wisdom and its ability to influence hormones such as FSH and AMH, moxibustion presents itself as an intriguing approach to fostering hormonal equilibrium. In the upcoming chapters, we will delve deeper into the potential effects of moxibustion in fertility enhancement and help individuals navigate a peaceful and well-balanced reproductive journey.

CHAPTER 4

Moxibustion and Ovarian Function: A deep dive into the impact of moxibustion on ovarian function.

Moxibustion has become well-known in the field of traditional Chinese medicine as a potent therapeutic method that can affect many facets of health and wellbeing. We will explore the substantial effects of moxibustion on ovarian function in this chapter, providing insight into how this traditional medicine may benefit women who are trying to become more fertile by promoting ovarian health, follicular development, and ovulation.

Reproductive Health and Ovarian Function:

The foundation of female reproductive health is ovarian function. The menstrual cycle, follicular development, ovulation, and hormonal balance are all regulated by the ovaries through their intricate interactions with various hormones and physiological processes. Anovulation, or insufficient ovulation, irregular menstrual periods, and difficulties with conception can result from disturbances in ovarian function. Moxibustion is a comprehensive method designed to optimize the complex functioning of the ovaries and bring them back into equilibrium.

Moxibustion's Mechanism on Ovarian Function:

Because moxibustion can improve blood circulation, stimulate Qi (qi flow), and balance Yin and Yang energies in the body, it has an impact on ovarian function. Moxibustion produces deep-penetrating localized heat at particular acupuncture points, which encourages vasodilation and increases blood flow to the ovaries. Improved follicular development, ovarian tissue nourishment, and good ovulation can all be attributed to this increased blood circulation.

Improving the Health of Ovaries:

The effects of moxibustion on ovarian health are complex. It can aid in the treatment of ailments including decreased ovarian reserve and polycystic ovary syndrome (PCOS), both of which have a detrimental effect on fertility.

1. PCOS (polycystic ovarian syndrome): Hormonal abnormalities and enlarged ovaries

with many cysts are two hallmarks of PCOS. Ovulatory function can be restored and cyst formation can be decreased with the use of moxibustion's capacity to control hormone levels and increase blood flow to the ovaries. Indirect moxibustion in particular helps balance hormones without producing excessive heat, which may be beneficial for those with PCOS.

2. Reduced Progenitor Reserve (PRR): When a mother ages, her ovaries produce fewer eggs, both in terms of quantity and quality. This

condition is known as delayed ovulation (DOR). The ability of moxibustion to increase blood flow to the ovaries may help to improve the microenvironment required for the production of follicles. Frequent moxibustion treatments may improve ovarian response and egg quality.

Ovulation and Follicle Development:

For ovulation and conception to be successful, ovarian follicles must mature and release an egg through a process known as follicular development. Affected by moxibustion in this procedure are:

1. Encouraging Follicle Development: Moxibustion's increased blood circulation can help grow follicles by facilitating the supply of nutrients and oxygen. This food promotes their development and maturation, which raises the possibility of a successful ovulation.

2. Supporting Ovulation: The effects of moxibustion on ovarian blood flow and hormonal balance can foster an ideal ovulation

environment. Moxibustion promotes appropriate connection between the brain and ovaries, which aids in the release of a mature egg.

Attailing Moxibustion to Health of the Ovarian:

Suitability of moxibustion for improving ovarian function depends on individualised treatment protocols. An experienced practitioner selects the right acupuncture sites and moxibustion procedures based on the patient's diagnosis, menstruation history, and general health.

1. Acupuncture Point Selection: Moxibustion treatments for ovarian health frequently target acupuncture points associated to the ovaries, such as Ren-4 (Guan Yuan) and Ren-3 (Zhong Ji). It is thought that these sites support follicular development, balance menstrual cycles, and nourish the ovaries.

2. Chemical Combustion Rate: The number of moxibustion sessions is determined by the demands of each

individual. In order to ensure constant ovarian function, more frequent treatments may be advised for individuals with irregular menstrual cycles or hormonal abnormalities.

3. Limited Treatments: Moxibustion can be combined with other traditional Chinese medical practices, such acupuncture and herbal therapy, to improve fertility in a holistic way.

Rendering:

The possibility that moxibustion can improve ovarian function gives those who are struggling with infertility hope. For the best ovarian health, follicular growth, and ovulation, moxibustion promotes hormonal balance, energy flow harmony, and blood circulation. As with any therapeutic intervention, it is important to speak with a trained professional who can customize moxibustion treatments to meet individual requirements and help people on their path to better reproductive health and well-being.

CHAPTER 5

Managing PCOS (Polycystic Ovary Syndrome) with Moxibustion: Focus on how moxibustion can be used as a complementary therapy for individuals with PCOS. Explore its potential benefits in addressing insulin resistance, hormonal imbalances, and other

aspects of PCOS-related fertility challenges.

The complicated endocrine condition known as polycystic ovarian syndrome, or PCOS, affects millions of people globally and poses a number of risks to reproductive health. Interest in alternative and holistic methods of treating PCOS symptoms and related fertility problems has increased as the condition's prevalence rises. This chapter explores the relationship between PCOS and moxibustion, shedding light on the possible advantages of moxibustion as a supplemental treatment for those facing infertility issues associated with PCOS.

Comprehensing PCOS: An Endocrine Mysterium:

Many symptoms, such as irregular menstrual cycles, ovarian cysts, hormonal abnormalities, and frequently insulin resistance, are indicative of polycystic ovary syndrome (PCOS). These complex circumstances might cause problems with ovulation and conception, which can be quite difficult for people who want to become parents.

As a method based on fostering equilibrium among the body's energy systems, moxibustion has the capacity to treat multiple aspects of PCOS, providing a comprehensive strategy that goes beyond treating symptoms.

Dressing Insulin Resistance: An Important Suggested Piece:

One of the main characteristics of PCOS is insulin resistance, which also leads to metabolic disturbances and hormone abnormalities. It has been investigated whether moxibustion applied at particular acupuncture locations could regulate insulin sensitivity. Moxibustion is believed to produce localized heat that improves blood circulation, which may facilitate the body's absorption of glucose and increase insulin sensitivity.

Although investigations investigating the precise effect of moxibustion on insulin resistance in PCOS are still under progress, preliminary results indicate that moxibustion may provide a useful adjunctive approach for handling this significant facet of PCOS-associated reproductive difficulties.

Moxibustion and Hormone Harmonization:

Elevated androgen (male hormone) levels and abnormal hormone signaling are common features of PCOS. In the setting of PCOS, the ability of moxibustion to modify hormonal balance assumes further significance. Moxibustion modifies acupuncture sites linked to hormone regulation in an effort to bring the endocrine system back into balance.

Promising research has been done on how moxibustion affects hormone levels in PCOS patients. Moxibustion may affect hormone levels, which could lead to more regular menstrual periods and better ovulatory function, according to studies.

Beyond Symptom Management: An All-encompassing Method:

Beyond only treating symptoms, moxibustion's holistic approach aims to bring the body back into balance. Moxibustion may help with stress reduction, relaxation, and general well-being in addition to treating insulin resistance and hormone imbalances. This all-encompassing strategy is in line with the complex nature of PCOS and how it affects fertility.

Participatory Care: Combining Moxibustion with PCOS Treatment:

Notable is the potential for moxibustion to supplement traditional medical approaches to PCOS care. It is recommended that people with PCOS collaborate with medical specialists to create an integrative care plan that includes moxibustion in addition to other therapies including dietary changes, exercise, and medication if needed.

In summary:

Within the complex field of PCOS-related reproductive difficulties, moxibustion presents itself as a potent means of comprehensive care. By addressing hormonal imbalances, insulin resistance, and other larger aspects of well-being, moxibustion provides PCOS patients with a comprehensive strategy to controlling their illness and improving fertility. Later chapters will explore more aspects of moxibustion's effects and help readers navigate a more peaceful and empowered reproductive path as we dig deeper into the practice's

possible uses in the field of
fertility.

CHAPTER 6

Moxibustion Protocols for Different Phases of the Menstrual Cycle: Provide detailed guidance on using moxibustion at different stages of the menstrual cycle, including menstruation, follicular phase, ovulation, and luteal phase. Discuss specific points and techniques for each phase.

Understanding the various phases of the menstrual cycle in detail is necessary in order to fully utilize moxibustion's ability to improve fertility. We will examine specific moxibustion procedures for the luteal phase, ovulation, follicular phase, and menstrual cycle in this chapter. By focusing on particular acupuncture sites and using the right methods, people can improve their reproductive health and raise their chances of becoming pregnant.

Period of Menstruation: Fostering Rebirth

The body goes through a process of regeneration and shedding during menstruation. Moxibustion encourages mild warmth and circulation to the pelvic region, which can assist this natural cycle.

Points of Acupuncture: - Ren-4 (Guan Yuan): This location, which is beneath the navel, is thought to support the uterus during menstruation and nourish the reproductive organs.

The technique involves using an indirect moxibustion method by holding a moxa roll or stick above Ren-4.

- Use the warmth for fifteen to twenty minutes to encourage circulation and relaxation.

Nourishing Follicles: Follicular Phase

When ovarian follicles grow and mature, it is known as the follicular phase. Moxibustion can enhance follicular development and improve blood supply to the ovaries during this stage.

Points of Acupuncture: - Ren-4 (Guan Yuan) and Ren-3 (Zhong Ji): These sites support ovarian nourishment and menstrual cycle regulation.

Combining direct and indirect moxibustion procedures is the technique.
- To encourage blood flow to the ovaries, use indirect moxibustion to Ren-3 and Ren-4 and direct moxibustion using a moxa cone on

important acupuncture points such as SP-6 (San Yin Jiao).

Stage of Ovulation: Encouraging Release

The release of a developed egg from the ovary is known as ovulation. During this stage, moxibustion can assist the hormonal shifts and help with the ovulatory process.

Acupuncture Points: - SP-6 (San Yin Jiao): This point is utilized for improving blood flow to the reproductive organs and controlling menstrual periods.

- CV-4 (Guan Yuan) and CV-3 (Zhong Ji): These locations facilitate a smooth ovulatory process and support the ovaries.

Technique: - To enhance circulation and hormonal balance, use indirect moxibustion on SP-6, CV-3, and CV-4.

- To avoid overheating, concentrate on gradual warming methods.

Luteal Phase: Feeding the Luteum Corpus

The corpus luteum, which develops after ovulation and secretes progesterone to prime the uterine lining for possible implantation, is what defines the luteal phase.

Acupressure Points: - Zhong Ji at CV-3 and Guan Yuan at CV-4: Support is still offered by these locations during the luteal phase.

- Qi Hai, Ren-6: This point helps to nourish the uterus and maintain the lining of the uterus.

The approach involves using a blend of direct and indirect moxibustion methods to the assigned acupuncture points.
The corpus luteum and the uterine lining should be supported by focusing on preserving a loving and balanced warmth.

Combining Moxibustion with the Entire Cycle:

The whole menstrual cycle can benefit from the application of moxibustion for a more thorough approach. Tailored moxibustion techniques can improve the menstrual cycle's inherent rhythm, meet particular demands, and foster a positive environment for conception.

Conclusion

One useful method for enhancing every stage of the menstrual cycle is moxibustion. Acupuncture treatments that target particular acupuncture sites can help people achieve reproductive system harmony, promote hcalthy follicular development, and facilitate smooth ovulation. To ensure a well-rounded and successful approach to fertility enhancement, it is imperative to obtain advice from a qualified and experienced practitioner who can customize moxibustion protocols to meet the needs of each individual.

CHAPTER 7

Self-Care and Moxibustion Practices at Home: Empower readers to incorporate moxibustion into their daily routine for fertility enhancement. Offer practical tips and step-by-step instructions for safe and effective self-administration of moxibustion at home.

The importance of self-care in the quest for enhanced fertility cannot be emphasized. As people assume greater responsibility for their health and want to maximize their reproductive potential, it is critical to include holistic practices into everyday life. With its extensive history and possible advantages, moxibustion presents a special kind of self-care that may be used in the convenience of one's own home. By providing readers with the information and useful tools they need to smoothly integrate moxibustion into their daily routines, this chapter supports their sense of agency and well-being as they pursue conception.

Accepting the Sanctuary at Home:

A caring environment in the house is necessary for self-care routines to be successful. Before going into the details of moxibustion, advise readers to create a peaceful area in which they may unwind and find their core. To further improve this setting and create a haven for self-healing, add aromatherapy, soft lighting, and relaxing music.

Introducing Yourself to Moxa:

Introduce readers to moxa, the mainstay of moxibustion therapy, first. Describe the various kinds of moxa that are available, such as the stick, cone, and smokeless kinds. Describe the preparation procedure for moxa and stress the need of choosing premium moxa for secure and efficient use.

Choosing Points of Acupuncture:

Give advice on which acupuncture points to use for improving conception. These points may be used to stimulate relaxation, control hormones, and target the reproductive organs. Provide readers with images or diagrams to assist them in locating these spots on their own bodies.

Effective and Safe Moxibustion Methods:

Take readers through the self-administering moxibustion procedure step-by-step. In order to avoid burns or discomfort, emphasize safety precautions while highlighting both direct and indirect techniques. Describe the significance of keeping a proper distance from the skin and how to modify the moxibustion's duration according to each person's comfort level.

Rates and Timing:

Talk about when and how often moxibustion sessions are best. Take into account elements including personal schedules, overall objectives, and the menstrual cycle. I would advise readers to create a regimen that they stick to, whether it is weekly, daily, or timed to correspond with particular menstrual cycles.

Inhalation and Awareness:

Incorporate breathing exercises and mindfulness into your moxibustion routines. Lead readers through techniques for deep breathing that will improve their ability to relax and focus their good energy. Stress the relationship between the mind and body and invite readers to practice mindfulness during moxibustion sessions.

Notes and Contemplation:

It is recommended that readers keep a moxibustion notebook in order to document their feelings, experiences, and observations. A journal gives people a place to reflect on themselves, which enables them to see how they're doing and modify their self-care routines accordingly.

Looking for Expert Advice:

Although practicing self-care at home can be empowering, it's crucial to get advice from a licensed healthcare provider. A certified acupuncturist or TCM practitioner should be consulted by individuals to make sure that moxibustion techniques meet their unique needs and objectives.

The incorporation of moxibustion into self-care routines presents a special chance for people to actively participate in their well-being on the path to fertility improvement. Incorporating moxibustion into everyday life is made easier for readers by this chapter's practical advice and confidence-boosting techniques. As more people come to understand how moxibustion may be a transformational tool in their own house, upcoming chapters will explore how self-care practices can complement more comprehensive fertility enhancement techniques.

CHAPTER 8

Combining Moxibustion with Other Holistic Approaches: Explore synergies between moxibustion and other holistic practices such as acupuncture, herbal medicine, meditation, and dietary modifications. Discuss how a comprehensive approach can optimize fertility outcomes.

Enhancing fertility is a complex process that can be considerably improved by taking a comprehensive strategy. This chapter will examine the potent synergies that result from combining moxibustion with various holistic therapies such herbal medicine, meditation, acupuncture, and dietary adjustments. People can enhance their reproductive outcomes and provide a harmonious foundation for conception by adopting a complete plan.

1. Harmonizing Energy with Acupuncture and Moxibustion

Combining moxibustion and acupuncture can provide additional benefits as they both have roots in traditional Chinese medicine. Moxibustion uses heat to increase Qi flow, whereas acupuncture uses tiny needles inserted into predetermined locations to balance the body's energy (Qi). As a group, they can:

Improve Blood Flow: The heat of moxibustion encourages blood circulation, and the needles of acupuncture boost energy and blood flow. This mixture supports the health and function of reproductive organs by enhancing the flow of nutrients and oxygen to them.

- Regulate Hormones: The menstrual cycle and fertility can benefit from hormonal balance, which is facilitated by moxibustion's ability to harmonize Yin and Yang energies and acupuncture's effect on the endocrine system.

2. Moxibustion and Herbal Medicine: Caring from Within

Traditional medicinal procedures have historically included both herbal medicine and moxibustion. Combining the two can provide a comprehensive external and internal strategy for enhancing fertility:

- Nutrition Within: Herbal treatments can be customized to treat particular imbalances or illnesses that impact fertility. In concert with moxibustion, they maintain the body's internal systems continuously.

Auxiliary Stimulation: Herbal plasters or poultices can be used in conjunction with moxibustion's localized heat to maximize the therapeutic benefits of both techniques. For example, to enhance the effect of heat on particular places during moxibustion, a mixture of warming herbs can be administered topically.

3. Moxibustion and Meditation: Fostering a Mind-Body Bond

By balancing the mind and body, meditation, mindfulness, and relaxation techniques can create an atmosphere that is favorable to conception. In conjunction with moxibustion:

Reduction of Stress: The calming warmth of moxibustion combines with the calming effects of meditation to reduce stress hormones that may have an adverse effect on fertility.

Psycho-Somatic Link: People who meditate are better able to connect with their bodies and intuition needs. This awareness can help patients feel more deeply connected to the benefits of moxibustion, which can increase its efficacy.

4. Nutritional Adjustments and Moxibustion: Feeding the Basis

Food has a big impact on fertility, and you can maximize your body's reproductive health by combining moxibustion with dietary changes:

- Dietary Assistance: A dict high in nutrients and well-balanced helps support reproduction. The effects of moxibustion on digestion can improve the body's absorption of nutrients, guaranteeing that it gets the building blocks it needs for reproduction.

Digestive Harmony: By enhancing effective digestion and absorption of nutrients crucial for reproductive health, moxibustion's stimulation of digestive acupoints can support dietary adjustments.

Developing an All-Inclusive Fertility Plan:

Combining moxibustion with other holistic methods creates a complete reproductive plan that takes into account the person's emotional, physical, and energy needs. A holistic approach, by customizing each modality to the unique requirements of the individual, can:

- Maximize Health of Reproduction: When many techniques are integrated, the body's internal milieu is nurtured, hormones are balanced, and blood flow is improved—all of which provide an ideal condition for conception.

- Promote Emotional Health: In order to promote emotional resilience and lessen worry, holistic therapies frequently incorporate mindfulness and stress-reduction methods. These can have a good impact on the results of conception.

- Promote Body Awareness: The holistic approach helps people become more aware of their bodies, empowering them to take an active role in their reproductive process.

Rendering:

Combining moxibustion with other holistic techniques results in a synergistic dance that profoundly connects with the body's innate intelligence. Through the use of acupuncture, herbal medicine, meditation, and dietary adjustments, people can optimize the results of their fertility journey. This all-encompassing approach recognizes the body, mind, and spirit as being interconnected and encourages people in the direction of a harmonious, balanced route to conception and improved wellbeing.

www.ingramcontent.com/pod-product-compliance
Lightning Source LLC
Chambersburg PA
CBHW050738260726
48661CB00001B/292